Only your Hairstylist Knows...

...until now!

∾

Judy Gagleard

Contents

Introduction

Without sounding like an actor giving an Academy Award speech, I would like to acknowledge all of the hardworking, caring, beautiful, and talented hairstylists who have worked diligently in order to master the craft. Hairstylists listen to their clients' stories on a daily basis. We smile, nod our heads, and respond to many different clients who love to vent to their hairstylists. Unfortunately, we stand behind our styling chairs for hours a day. The passion we have for our profession outweighs the physical inconveniences we have to endure.

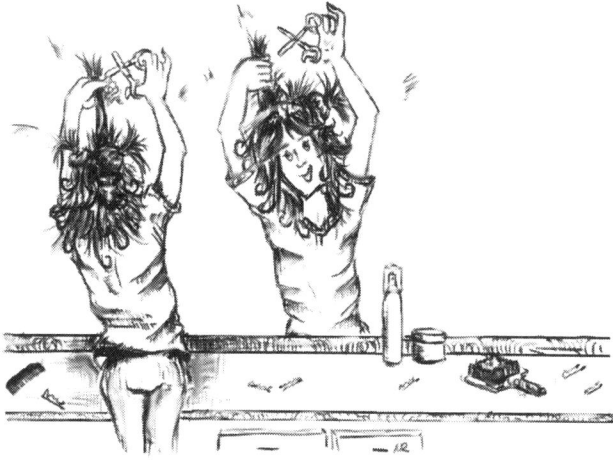

I Just Want to be a Hairstylist

What are the early signs that a little girl will grow up to be a professional hairstylist?

At a very early age, I would braid my sister's hair. I would style, comb, and brush their hair. The babysitter could not believe a five-year-old could braid hair. I was cutting my sister's hair and bangs at the same age, but their bangs always looked like a five-year-old had cut them.

My mother was furious after the first time I cut my sister's hair and my own. My sisters and I always wore our hair in pigtails. I told my younger sister, Jackie, that if she let me cut her pigtail off and bury it in the dirt that it would grow faster. She must have agreed with me because I cut her hair right to the rubber band near her scalp.

After the rubber band fell to the ground, Jackie ran into the house to look at her hair. When I heard her cry to my mom, I knew she was looking in the mirror.

I just sat down on our front porch and waited for my mom to come running out of the house to ask me what I had done to my sister's hair. She started to yell at me until she looked at what I had also done to my own hair. Lucky for me, my mom had a great sense of humor. She started to laugh uncontrollably. She grabbed the kitchen scissors from my hands before I caused any more damage.

I told her why I cut our hair. She just stood in front of me and said, "Please do not ever try to make your hair or your sister's hair grow faster again."

We decided to let nature take care of that.

I believe I started the shag hair style before it was popular. There is a technique where you put the hair into a ponytail and then cut the hair around the rubber band area. This technique cuts the top layer shorter than the other layers. The layers continue to be longer as the hair falls.

My other sister, Roxanne, never let me cut her hair until she was in the seventh grade. I still remember standing in my Aunt Irma's bathroom, cousin Mona handing me the kitchen scissors to cut my sister's bangs. My cousin was always with me and my sisters to assist us in any mischievous maneuvers. Mona knew I loved to style anybody's hair if they would allow me to.

It felt like my lucky day when she handed me the kitchen scissors and said, "Judy, you have more practice than anyone else in this house when it comes to cutting hair."

I turned to my sister with a huge smile on my face and wide open eyes. I couldn't wait to master cutting bangs. My sister was very confident with my styling skills, but I had never cut her bangs before. Roxanne was talking as I started to cut her bangs right at her eyebrow. She claimed the scissors nipped her forehead. To this day, I still believe they just grazed her skin.

She started to yell, "You cut me!"

I turned her to the mirror and asked, "Do you see any blood?"

She said, "No, but that scared me. I could feel the sharpness of the scissors."

I thought I would be very careful and pull the bangs down to finish the cut. To my surprise, I found out the hard way what happens when you comb the hair down flat on to the forehead. It makes the hair appear longer than it actually is.

When I cut the other side of her bangs even with the side I had already cut, the hair sprung up to the middle of her forehead as soon as I released it from my grasp. I was only in the sixth grade. How was I supposed to know that I used two different techniques on her bangs? One look at my face, and Roxanne asked me what was wrong.

I asked her if she had a headband with her because she might want to wear it today.

She looked into the mirror and started to scream at me. "What have you done to my bangs?"

I was so shocked myself that I could not even respond.

The worst part of this story was that it was picture day at school. Oh yes! We still have the picture to remind us of this episode. My sister was very popular in school. I knew that whatever she did with her hair, everyone else would approve of her choice. She was only five feet tall and weighed about one hundred pounds with beautiful light red hair.

After I calmed her down, I parted her hair from one side to the other to cover her forehead and shorter bang area. She never let me forget that day.

Another story that my brother-in-law, Ron Gill, loves to tell is about the first time I cut his hair. He has been married to Roxanne for over thirty years now. Ron went to school with my family in Canton. We were friends with him in high school where Roxanne met Ron. He is known as one of the funniest guys in Canton.

Ron visited our house frequently when we were in high school. My three sisters and a brother always had many of our friends and relatives at the house at the same time. My cousin, Mary Margaret Lee Campbell, was one of our closest cousins who seemed more like a sister to all of us. My sisters and I were either at her house after school, or she would be at our house. This is why Ron always visited our house after he worked on his dad's farm: he knew there would be plenty of girls to joke around with him.

One day Ron came over after he had gone to the barber to get his hair cut. I took one look at him and started to laugh. He asked me what was so funny. I told him that one of his ears was lower than the other. He looked in the mirror and saw one of his ears covered with hair while the other ear was totally bare. He didn't notice the horrible haircut he had just received from the barber shop. Without even asking him if I could cut his hair, I went into the kitchen to get the scissors and balanced his haircut for him.

Ron has never gone back to a barber shop after that incident. He has been my client for over thirty-eight years. Before I attended beauty college, Ron was my first non-related client. The first haircut that I gave him was with scissors, not a clipper. His style has changed since he was in high school. The color has now changed from a blonde color to a magnificent white color.

Jeff Horton is another of my brothers-in-law. Everybody knew Jeff Horton in school. He had suburb athletic abilities and was involved in all of the sports his high school provided. Our family consisted of five children as did the Horton family. Sam and Karen Horton had four boys, Michael, Curtis, Jeff and John and one girl named Kathy. They were all hot. They are still hot in their prime. They are not as hot as my husband, of course, but close.

Jeff was my first ear slip-up. It sounds painful, but Jeff claims he didn't feel anything. I had such a passion for cutting hair that I would carry my scissors in my purse with me at all times. These were professional scissors, not the kitchen scissors I used to cut Ron's hair with back in high school.

Jeff was just starting his plumbing business and never had time to get his hair cut at a barber shop. I offered to cut his hair at his and Jackie's house. I sat him in a chair that was not a professional salon chair. We were talking and having a good time, and I just clipped the very tip of his ear. It wasn't a bad cut, but it was just enough to draw blood. Jackie was right there to apply an ointment and stop the bleeding. I felt really bad because I had never cut any of my client's ears before. I don't think my sister believed me, but it was true.

Jeff was so cool about it. He told me not to worry. He was actually glad that my first injury was to him and not a paying client. I learned a lesson from my family members at an early stage of my career: relatives will keep coming back to you for a haircut, even if it is painful.

Every stylist has a story…

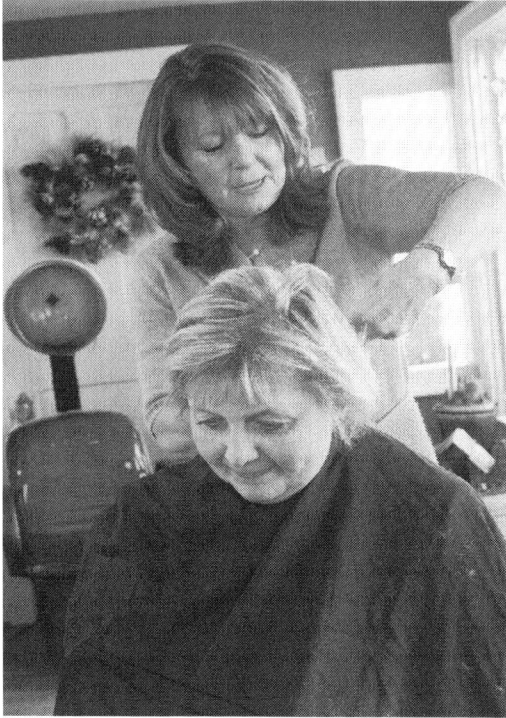

Chapter 2

A Day in the Life of a Hairstylist

Stylists listen to stories about the most important part of the clients' day during their salon visit. When the stylist's schedule on the appointment book consists of five clients, the stylist may hear five totally different stories from each individual client. If the stylist's schedule consists of ten clients, then the stylist will hear ten different stories. I don't know many women who wouldn't enjoy talking to five to ten different women every day about their concerns. This time and opportunity to vent about a husband or children in the stylist's chair is more economical than therapy, and it comes with a great hair style, too.

When my girls were growing up, I enjoyed repeating my happy stories about them to all of my clients. I thought my clients were as excited as I was to hear about their every move and accomplishment. The regular clients usually liked to hear about my children as I liked to hear about their children. On the other hand, there are the clients who could care less about what stylists have to say and only want to talk about their own lives. If the stylist is lucky enough to have an opportunity to talk about his or her own life to the clients, then the stylist takes full advantage of that opportunity. As all of my clients and friends will attest, I have the gift of gab. Just imagine telling clients your favorite story over and over as each individual client sits in your chair throughout the day. While this is highly enjoyable for a stylist, co-workers get tired of hearing the same stories over and over again.

I feel blessed to have a profession that is also my passion. When you love what you do, you also feel like you have not worked a day in your life. This is how I have felt working as a hairstylist for over thirty years. My dreams will have come true if at least one of my stories has put a smile on my readers face or enlightened any of you in some way.

The salon atmosphere is usually a very positive and pleasant feeling. When a room consists of mostly women, it is full of laughter and conversations; women usually enjoy listening to each other's point of view on an array of subjects. The clients also like to give advice, even if the stylist doesn't really want to hear it. They ask questions, give advice, and communicate, as only women can.

My one and only confrontation with a client was with an army sergeant who wanted a flat top with a clipper-cut. He didn't like how I cut his hair at all. My sister-in-law, Carol, and I were working at the same salon in Plymouth, Michigan. She had heard my client complaining to me about the sides of his hair, and she rescued me. She knew just what he wanted and could cut hair with clippers like no other stylist could. Carol finished his flat top haircut to perfection.

Professional people in all sorts of trades have their own techniques to accomplish any task requested with slightly different results. This man obviously didn't care for my technique. Carol knew he was happy with the final result because he gave her a twenty dollar tip. This was the biggest tip Carol had ever received from a client. I can still picture the look on her face when she realized she was holding a twenty dollar bill.

He then walked over to me and gave me a ten dollar tip with an apology for talking so rudely to me. He explained that he was a very important sergeant, and his men looked up to him. He told me that he had an image to maintain and would have felt embarrassed if he didn't have the exact hair cut every time. I told him that he needed to go to the same hairstylist in order to maintain his haircut. Unfortunately, neither Carol nor I ever had the pleasure of cutting "Mr. Exact's" hair again.

Listening to clients tell stories about their lives is a large part of what I do as a hairstylist. People have fun and interesting stories to tell on a daily basis, and people love to tell their hairstylist about their lives. I have been listening to people talk about their lives for over thirty years as a hairstylist.

"Only your hairstylist knows" is a phrase people use because so many people love to tell their hairstylist stories that they would never tell other people. The happy times and sad times are also in the stories that people tell. Clients enjoy having the stylist cut and style their hair because it is very pampering. Most people feel really comfortable talking to their stylist. We see clients every six weeks. In that time frame, we can usually share our life stories.

Clients have the sole attention of one person. It's not like going to the dentist or the doctor where the client is afraid of hearing bad news about their health. It's usually all positive, comfortable, and pleasant conversation. Clients can talk the whole session if the stylist is a good listener. The stylist isn't probing at you. No instrument is stuck in your mouth while you are trying to answer questions.

A professional hairstylist has the ability to read the clients. From the first eye contact that is made at the time of the appointment, to the consultation at the stylist's chair. For example, one client is a happy, perky person with positive stories. This client may talk to the stylist as soon as the stylist makes contact at the front desk. This type of client may not even take a breath to let the stylist know what hair style they would like to receive. The happy client is my favorite client because I love to hear about my clients' individual lives. I already know what I have to say, and so I want to hear what the client has to say.

The next client may not even want to look in the stylist's eyes when approached, looking at the floor as if they feel uncomfortable talking to new acquaintances. Normally this type of client is not interested in your personal business. I would try to read this person's response to my normal every day conversations. When I only hear a yes or no response to my questions, then I try to leave Miss Gabby in the backroom. I honestly have a hard time with this type of client. If I can't start a conversation with a client, it is obvious to me that this person has a very shy personality. I let them set the tone for the visit. My clients can attest that I don't like a non-verbal visit. However, I do respect the client's personality and have grown to respect their silence. I'm quite sure there are stylists who have lost a client over the nuisance of the gift of gab. I believe the gift of gab is a talent, not a nuisance.

The client should control the conversation instead of the stylist. There are clients who see only the bad side of every situation. These clients usually like to talk throughout the whole appointment. When the client chooses to talk and not listen then this sets the tone for the appointment. I usually let these clients talk out their frustrations. As hairstylists, we need to read our clients to know when to let them control the conversation. If the client wants to vent to the stylist, the professional stylists need to notice this and just listen to the paying client's concerns.

Communication is a strong asset for people in this profession. If the stylist doesn't know what the client is talking about, how can we give clients the service they expect and deserve? When a client asks me to cut one inch from their hair, I like to show them where their hair will fall after I make the cut. One piece of information I have learned is that not everyone's measurement is the same. Stylists can cut a half of an inch off of your client's hair and they might think that is too short. Another client would tell you to cut one inch or more off, and after you cut the length the client has asked you to cut, it is still not enough. This is part of the craft of being a hairstylist.

Many people complain about the hairstylist who doesn't listen to their explanations of what style they are trying to convey. Clients have talked about how frustrated they become when they ask for a slight trim and walk out of the salon with a style much shorter than what they were expecting. Pictures of the style and length are the best way to communicate with your stylist. Some clients bring in several different pictures with different frontal views in order to show the stylist what they cannot explain to them.

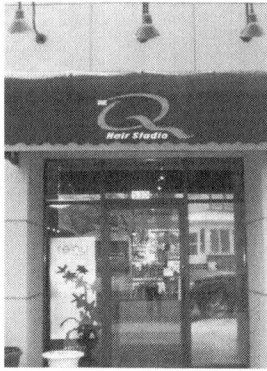

Most people can't wait to go to their favorite salon because of the refreshed feeling upon leaving after a new haircut. The majority of clients look so much better when they leave than when they arrived. Isn't this the reason some clients love their hairstylist?

෩

Each and every day, working in a salon is a totally unpredictable experience. Stylists have different appointments every day, and the stylists never know who just might be scheduled for an appointment on a daily basis. I remember always looking for Richard Gere or Tom Cruise's name on my appointment book. After waiting for three decades for one of these hot actors to book an appointment with me, I have finally given up on that fantasy.

It is exhilarating as a stylist to look at the daily appointment book to see familiar names on your schedule. The regular clients are like family members to me. I enjoy listening to their stories about their everyday lives. It's amazing how some clients have similar personalities. The different personalities are what keep this profession so alive.

When stylists are new to a salon, they never know from day to day whose hair they will be working on. I enjoy the challenge of meeting new clients and working with them to figure out what service they were interested in on that particular appointment. That type of connection with a total stranger is one of the most rewarding aspects of my career. I have had clients who don't really know what they are talking about when they are trying to explain a specific style to me, but I know exactly what they are talking about.

As a professional stylist with experience, the stylist's own techniques become a natural act to them. Clients are so thrilled when they feel like their stylist understands what they are trying to convey to the stylist. When the final results are just as the clients had imagined their hair would look, it is the best feeling in the world. The stylist knows they have accomplished a goal.

My family members are constantly telling me I have magic fingers after I style their hair. All I have to do is comb my fingers through their hair and magic begins. My three sisters and one brother claim I received all of the hairstyling talent in our family. They try to imitate my techniques but do not seem to get the same results.

I believe some stylists are naturals in their profession. The stylist can look at a haircut and, without even thinking about it twice, they know how to perform the style. Then there are other stylists, who are just doing their job. The client knows the difference in the stylist's work. A professional stylist's work is their craft. Stylists who are passionate about their craft will show that passion in their work.

My friend, Charlene Dunn, shared her story with me about a hairstylist who was not passionate about her craft.

A young girl worked part-time for Charlene's husband, Mike, at their family-owned roller skating rink. The girl asked Charlene if she could give her a body permanent wave on her already natural curly hair. The girl just finished beauty college and seemed to be quite talented, according to Charlene. The hairstylist said she was trained to work on all hair types, from straight to natural curly hair, while in school. My friend assumed the girl knew what she was doing. The girl was working at a salon at this time and asked my friend if she would come over to her house for the service instead of going into the salon. She agreed to go to her house only because she thought the girl would be much more comfortable in her own home than working in a salon.

The first request Charlene had for this girl was to make sure she only gave her a body perm and not a curly perm. My friend said she noticed the tiny perm rods that the girl intended to use and questioned their small size. The girl assured her she knew what she was doing and told my friend not to worry.

For the second time my friend told her how quickly and easily her hair would process a perm. Therefore she asked her not to leave the chemical solutions in her hair for a long period of time. After what seemed like forever, it was time to remove the perm rods from Charlene's hair. With the removal of each of the perm rods, her bob-length hair began to shrink. The hair was curlier and curlier as each perm rod was removed. My friend looked in the mirror to see how frizzy and dry her hair looked. She said it looked like she was wearing fur ear muffs over her ears.

The hairstylist never apologized for over-processing her hair. She didn't show any remorse for the poor service she had just given to a friend of hers. She then removed hair combs from her own hair and proceeded to comb my friend's hair back behind her ears using the decorative combs. The hairstylist told her she could keep the combs because she will need to wear them for a long time.

Eight months later, my friend was still trying to control her over-processed, permanent waved hair.

When I asked her why she thought this girl wanted to ruin her hair, she said, "This girl had a crush on my husband and wanted to make my hair look bad."

As a new hairstylist, you do learn from your mistakes. This profession has a unique result with each and every client who sits in your styling chair. While a particular process works for one client, it may not work on the next client. I strongly believe in asking a client what type of style they are not interested in achieving in order to master the style they are.

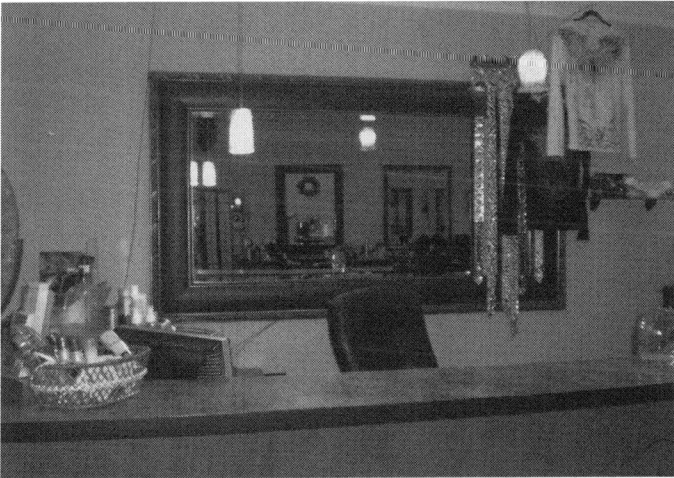

Chapter 3

Wait! The Receptionist Didn't Hear You

The receptionist is the first person the client will see when they enter the salon. This person needs to be well dressed, friendly, and professional. These traits are necessary in order to make a good first impression on the client. The first impression that is made by the receptionist sets the tone for the client's entire experience in the salon.

Only professional and very stylish people should apply for the receptionist position of a successful salon. This person should be wearing clothing that is appropriate for the salon environment. This could include a smock that coordinates with the colors of the salon. The receptionist's hair should always be styled and trendy. Their nails should be professionally manicured in order to present a polished look to the client.

A pleasant greeting as each client enters the salon is very important to provide a positive experience during the salon visit. Receptionist's desks are near the front of the salon in order to inform the stylist upon the client's arrival. The receptionist also answers questions, offers refreshments or gives the location of the salon's restrooms or coat closet, if the client chooses to hang their own coat in the provided closet.

They provide a service to the client that is necessary to the functionality of the salon. An example of a professional service provided by the receptionist could include walking a new client to the stylist and making introductions to make the client comfortable.

The receptionist should monitor when the stylist is ready for their next client. Informing the client of the wait time, and making suggestions to fill the time until the stylist is ready to begin the session is always a polite gesture. For example, the receptionist could explain any other services the salon has to offer and the price of these services.

The front desk should always be as neat as possible. No food should be in sight. Clients should not have to stand at the desk waiting for the receptionist to finish a last bite of lunch. The receptionist could have seasonal items, including food, to decorate the desk, but these decorations should be appropriate and tasteful.

൭൬

My favorite and most memorable receptionist's name was Cindy. She was the perfect person for the front entrance of a salon. Cindy had long vibrant red hair, big blue eyes, and her personality was even more vibrant than her hair. She was always in a good mood. Nobody was a stranger to Cindy. All of the clients adored her, as she adored them.

I can still envision Cindy looking over the receptionist desk in order to see what my client and I were doing. She would listen to the majority of the conversations between my clients and me. If she was interested in our conversation, she would call across the salon to ask us to wait for her to join our conversation.

Those were the days when I could remember any joke I heard. Cindy and I came up with a few regular jokes that we would share with new clients. If the client started to tell a joke and Cindy heard the beginning of it she would again lean over the desk and call for us to wait for her presence to continue.

The clients and other stylists would complain because the anticipation of the punch line of the joke was just killing them. We would laugh and tell Cindy she needed to get her cosmetology license to be on the floor when someone was telling a joke.

One of our favorite jokes was about an older woman who would approach a young girl, dining alone, at a restaurant.

The woman said, "You look just like my daughter. She moved out of state recently for a new job. I have cried myself to sleep every night since she left."

This made the girl feel really bad.

The woman asked, "Would you wave goodbye and call me 'Mom' when I go up to pay for my lunch? It would make me feel so much better. I haven't been called 'Mom' in such a long time."

The girl thought this was a strange request, but she told the woman that she would do this.

The woman took her bill up to the cashier, and turned around to wave at the young girl.

The girl called, "Bye, Mom!" She felt so good after helping a stranger. This good feeling only lasted until she approached the cashier to pay her own bill. Her bill was double the amount it should have been! When she told the cashier that her bill was wrong, the cashier looked at her as if she was being rude.

"There are two people on this bill. Your lunch and your mom's," the cashier explained.

"What are you talking about? My mom is not in this restaurant," the young woman said.

The cashier said, "I heard you say good-bye to her and wave when she came up to present her bill.

The girl yelled at the cashier, "That woman is not my mom!" She turned around and saw the older woman getting into her car.

Either Cindy or I would finish the joke by saying, "The girl immediately ran outside into the parking lot and started pulling the older woman out of the car. She pulled her by her hair, just before she pulled her leg, just like I am pulling your leg."

Everyone in the salon roared with laughter every time we told that joke to a new client. These memories were just a small portion of the pleasures of working as a hairstylist in a salon.

On a daily basis, the conversations were female-oriented rather than male oriented. The main reason we talked about more female issues was because the clientele during the day hours was primarily female. The salon was made of two rows of salon stations. The stylists took turns leading the floor conversation.

During the majority of the day, each stylist and their clients had their own personal conversations. Cindy enjoyed listening to all of the different stories between the stylists and the clients. She would comment on what we talked about as we approached the desk. She had one ear on the phone receiver and the other ear was listening to the salon floor conversations. She showed an interest in every client who confided in her. Cindy wanted people to know how much she cared about their concerns. She listened to their stories and responded in positive ways.

We all have our good days and our bad days at work. One day I was working long hours and felt like every client was talking about their negative stories. I heard about confrontations among family members, how tired one client felt all day, and the last client was giving her entire medical history since 1970. Whenever my client starts talking about their bowels, I try to change the subject. If you are thinking, "Oh, nobody shares those stories with their stylists," I am telling you—they do. This type of story is a rare occurrence for me.

Just as my last client left the salon on this day, Cindy looked at me and said, "You did not listen to one word your last client said to you."

I looked up at her and asked her what she was talking about. She continued to tell me how I responded to all of the clients questions at the right time. I nodded my head at the right moment, I laughed at the appropriate time, but I still would not be able to tell her what the client was talking about.

Cindy could read me like a book. She knew if a subject did not interest me, I would listen and respond accordingly, but my heart and soul was not into the conversation for every client. I confessed to her that I can only hear about clients' bowel movements for so long before I go on autopilot. Cindy and I started to laugh about how our husbands like to talk about their bowel movements, and one bowel movement story a day is still more than we care to hear.

Chapter 4

Ballsy Backroom

Every salon has a backroom somewhere in the building facility. The stylists use this backroom to communicate with each other about their clients. A true professional will use the backroom to console another stylist about any concerns. I'm sure we have all heard a good confrontation between a stylist and her client at some time in our careers.

The backroom is full of supplies to use on the clients. Usually stylists can select from four or five different manufacturers who make their own hair colors, bleach, and perm solutions. I have found in a salon the owner usually has a favorite company to work with. That owner will carry more supplies from the favorite company's product line.

A full service salon has ample supplies in order for the stylists to complete a very comfortable and successful service. For example, perms need extra cotton to put around the clients' hairlines and end papers for wrapping hair around the curlers for a perm. These are just a few of the supplies which would be located in the backroom instead of stored at the hairstylist's station.

The backroom is also the room with a counter that is used to mix products. The hairstylist would obtain the appropriate bowl or bottle, depending on the service rendered. This leaves the big mess in the back area where the clients will not see it.

There is usually a washer and dryer in the backroom area. This allows the stylist to wash and dry used towels. This is a convenience for the salon employees. Hairstylists need towels for almost every service rendered. For example, the hairstylist puts a towel around each client's neck to protect the neck area from any chemical damage to the client's skin or clothing.

Stylists' faces show a look of relief each time they enter the backroom. It is not unusual to see a stylist roll her eyes because they cannot believe what just happened on the professional salon floor. In the backroom, stylists can express themselves in a way which might not seem appropriate around clients. The stylists can say what they really would like to say out on the salon floor. Clients should not be allowed to enter the backroom area of the salon. Truthfully, this is because stylists talk to each other about their clients. I'm not saying that all stylists gossip or have a potty mouth, but there are a few choice words uttered during the work day which are only appropriate for the backroom.

It is exhilarating to talk to the other co-workers about your accomplishments on the salon floor. We give great advice to each other and console each other in the backroom.

Occasionally stylists have heard about a little catfight which took place in the backroom. One person in particular was always trying to tell the other stylists what they should and should not do in and out of the backroom. This person asked me why I did not put away a bottle that was still sitting on the work counter. I told her I was not finished with my client, and I would put it away when I completed my service for my client.

Shortly after the confrontation with her, we crossed each other's path while entering the backroom. I looked straight into her eyes and said, "I think you should check your pants because I think you have balls in them."

She looked at me as if she had just seen a ghost. With fury in her eyes, she raised her hand to slap me across the face. I grabbed her hand while it was in mid-air and told her that if she wanted to have a good day, she had better put her attitude away. I then threw her hand away from me as I released it. She then started to cry and asked me to forgive her for being so rude. Naturally, I told her I would. I have never had a physical encounter with any co-worker, and I hope to God that I never do.

I explained to her how I felt about her confronting a co-worker on the salon floor in front of clients. The clients should never hear stylists' disagreements. I was in my twenties when this confrontation happened. I had an opinion on everything at that young age. Today I would never have used the same words of choice to express my frustrations. The ballsy stylist understood the message. We were friends for many years after this disagreement, until we drifted apart after she quit working at that salon many years later.

Most people do not expect their victim to respond to them during a confrontation. I, on the other hand, like to confront people who try to bully me or other co-workers during the attack. I enjoy thinking about the face on the bully when they realize they have bullied the wrong person.

Co-workers who talk about other people behind their backs all the time deserve to be confronted face to face by the person they are talking about. I have tried this method and it works. If I have a problem with a person I will confront them face to face with my situation, instead of spreading unnecessary gossip to other employees.

People who handle uncomfortable situations immediately have a peace about them. Arguments start when co-workers disagree with each other but are afraid to discuss their issues. I have always taken care of my issues right away and just feel this amazing relief. People who let issues linger for days just fester in their anger. The person who likes to bully others is usually very insecure. Bully's need to stop their vicious cycle.

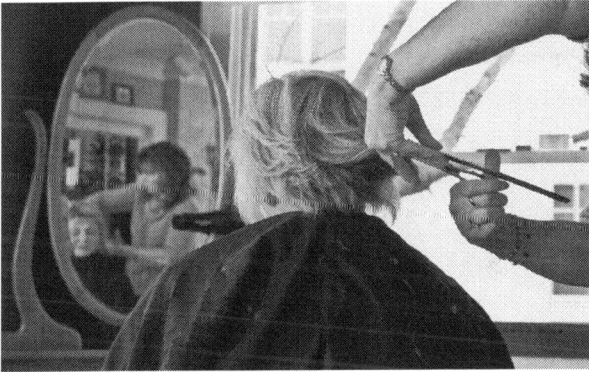

Chapter 5

Working at a Major Salon

What great memories I have from working as a stylist in a major salon! There were fifteen stylists who were hired for the grand opening of this new salon. I can still see the faces of each one of the stylists in my mind.

Two of the stylists became very good friends of mine. Their names are Agnes Hersey and Cindy Tollis. We are still very good friends and see each other whenever possible. We worked next to each other and talked to each other all day. Stylists become friends with the other stylists as well as their clients. Each stylist listens to the co-workers' conversations with their clients. We add our advice, even if they do not really want to hear it, to many conversations every day.

My friend Agnes was a very hard worker. She never left the salon to even go out to lunch. She booked her clients every fifteen minutes and had a great production line of clients. Agnes tried for years to convince Cindy and me to work through our lunch hours. We always crossed out the 12:00-1:00 spot on the scheduling book for lunch. That was my favorite hour of the day. It was fun to go into the mall and shop or eat a nice lunch with Cindy and other co-workers.

As many hairstylists know, if the stylist stops production, they will not make as much money as they would if one client was processing while starting a style on another.

Agnes made me realize that if I wanted to make a lot of money as a stylist, I needed to keep the production line going all day. She told me to eat my lunch in the backroom while my client was processing or in between other services.

It took many years before I took her great advice. I finally stopped blocking an hour from my schedule for lunch and replaced it with appointments. From that day forward my commission increased substantially on my paychecks. It also increased my weekly gross by adding those five hours to my week.

The three of us always helped each other with our clients. If Cindy needed her client's perm rinsed, either Agnes or I would gladly rinse it for her. We worked as a team, and it showed in our workmanship. When one of us went on vacation, the other two would team up and style the regular clients' hair for the stylist who was not available that week.

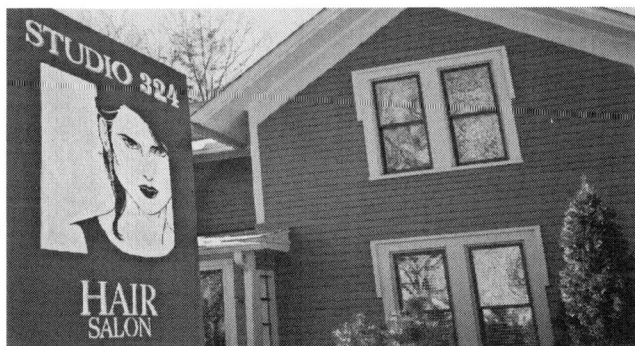

I believe a successful salon is a salon without drama. When the stylists enjoy each other's company and work well together, it makes the salon a pleasant place to visit for the clientele.

In the 80's, we booked up to three perms a day. Everyone wanted full hair or curly hair. The uniperm was the most popular perm of the decade. It had clamps on a tall, heated machine. After we wrapped our perms, we would put small clamps on the perm rod for just six minutes. It was ridiculous to think everyone would process in the same amount of time. The uniperm was popular for about five years, and then we realized how damaging it was to the hair. We went back to timing our perms for each client's hair.

In the 80's we also had weekly standing appointments for our clients to have their hair washed and styled. I know you can't believe that women did not wash their own hair like women do today. Even more bizarre is the fact that women only had their hair washed once a week. Oh yes. Washing your hair every day was not heard of for women who had standing appointments in a salon before the '90s.

I often wonder how the major product suppliers stayed in business. Women are all about using the correct product on their hair today. On a daily basis, or at least every other day, the majority of my clients now use a mousse, hair spray, and a third product that adds shine to their hair.

It is amazing how different the trends of hairstyles have changed through the years. Hair styles have changed from very straight hair in the 70's to very curly styles in the 80's and early 90's, and then back to straight hair again in the late 90's through the date of publication. My thirty years' experience as a hairstylist have seen many different hairstyles come and go.

Stylists usually work with five or more clients a

day. The majority of the clients are satisfied with the service rendered. They come in and are happy to just have someone style their hair. Then the day comes when a hairstylist will get a walk- in client who, no matter what the hairstylist does, the client will not be satisfied with the results.

I have seen stylists come into the backroom, crying, because a client didn't like the style or cut they received. The problem is usually a miscommunication between the stylist and the client.

There are going to be days when you just can't seem to please any client. Then there are other days when you seem to connect with every client.

Some clients are going to think you are great and other clients are not going to like your style. I have advised hairstylists to be confident in their own work. You will never please all of the clients all of the time.

Chapter 6

Pantyhose are Not Comfortable

There was a time when I thought everyone was just like me. If I woke up happy, then everyone should be happy. The rude awakening that this was not true came to me once I started working in a hair salon.

As a stylist, I try to read my clients. As I approach the front waiting area where the clients are waiting for their name to be called, I attempt to judge their mood. For example, I look to see if they are talking to other clients or sitting quietly waiting to hear their name called from the receptionist. Once the client is sitting at my station, I observe their demeanor again. I often wonder if they want to talk to me during the salon visit or if they want a quick style in order to get on with their daily life.

When I worked for a major salon, the stylists took classes about how to greet the clients. First impressions are a major factor when meeting a client. If the stylist doesn't look like they care about their own hair, then how are they going to care about the client's hair? Stylists are judged by their appearances during that first hello.

In the late 70's, hairstylists wore uniforms. Don't laugh; it made it very easy to get dressed in the morning. Each day was a different color of uniform, although some were hideous. One uniform was an ugly brown, and another one was yellow. Nothing looked good with either of them. It didn't matter what accessories were added. They were just plain and ugly.

I love the fact that now hairstylists can be stylish and wear trendy clothes to work in a salon. Most hairstylists are known for dressing with a lot of pizzazz. It makes me smile when I hear the comment, "You dress like a hairstylist." Stylists can dress in weird and quirky ways, and it is totally acceptable.

While working for a major salon when I was only in my twenties, the stylists were told that we had to wear dresses with high heeled shoes to work every day. We were no longer allowed to wear dress pants to work. The stylists were devastated by this change in policy. When hairstylists are standing in one position for six to eight hours a day, they need to wear comfortable shoes, not high-heeled dress shoes. In the 70's, they didn't make comfy shoes like they do now. Women who wore a dress and dress shoes, also wore pantyhose. I hope everyone reading this has heard of pantyhose. The young women today do not wear hosiery. Why didn't I come up with that trend years ago? I might have been on time everyday if I didn't have to fight with putting my pantyhose on. We also had to check each pair for a possible run in the toes or heel area.

The backroom was where all of the hairstylists vented about this dress code policy. We decided to talk to management and ask if there could be an exception to the new rule. Our boss tried to reason with her manager to no avail. The stylists were not pleased with the outcome of the management meeting.

All thirty stylists agreed to attend a meeting in order to plead our case. Only five of the thirty women had the courage to voice their opinion face-to-face with management. The worst part of this story was when we actually sat in the office with the top management to discuss our problem, not one of the other stylists would speak up. No one wanted to tell the boss how displeased they were with the new dress code, except for me. I told him we would not do a good job if we weren't comfortable in our clothing and shoes. We had worn nursing shoes all day, and now we were told we had to wear dress shoes. I looked at him with hope in my eyes that he would be sympathetic with our concerns. He shocked me when he told us about his grandma who wore pantyhose everyday and was comfortable in them. With an open mouth shocked look on my face I asked him how he, as a man, can tell us women that pantyhose are comfortable. I asked him if he had ever worn pantyhose for an entire work day. I then told him if you have never worn pantyhose, then how can you tell us they are comfortable? He looked at me as if he had just seen a ghost. His face turned a little red. I was not afraid to stand up for myself or my co-workers. He was talking about a subject he knew nothing about.

My boss intervened in the conversation by telling her manager to consider our concerns and get back with us. Our boss couldn't believe I had asked the manager of the store if he had ever worn pantyhose. I told her I was not going to back down just because he was my boss. He needed to know how we felt. In the end, we did leave our nursing shoes at our stations to wear during work hours only. We compromised by walking in and out of the salon in dress shoes.

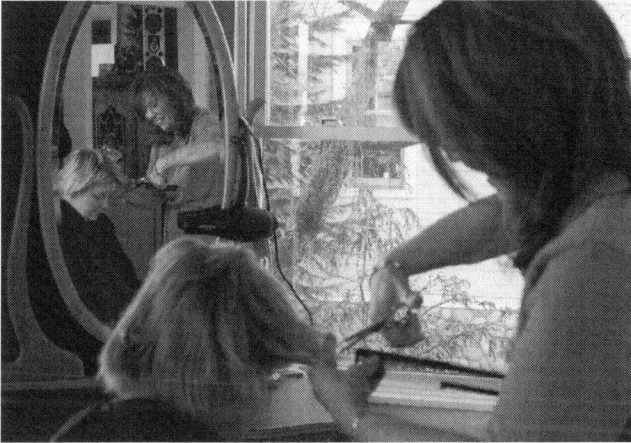

...until now! ⤴ 39

Chapter 7

Kill them with Kindness

The stories I am about to share are the rare stories that hairstylists do not hear in a salon every day. They are all true stories that I have experienced or that clients have shared with me.

The everyday experience in a salon is usually a very friendly, pleasant, and cordial experience. The normal conversations are about clients' families and everyday conversations. But a lot can happen in six weeks, between visits to the salon, to clients' and their families. We try to keep each other informed about our lives at each appointment. Each client has a different lifestyle and different opinions on many subjects.

When a client shares their insecurities with me, I always try to encourage them to be confident. A positive and confident attitude can turn an unpleasant situation into a pleasant situation. Hairstylists need to kill their clients with kindness. The cosmetology business is a very competitive business. Therefore, this is one way that stylists can get an edge over other stylists or other salons.

Through my years of experience, I have worked on clients who, at first glance, seem very uncomfortable with a new stylist cutting or coloring their hair. It is not a personal issue for me. This is when I kill my client with kindness. If the client is rude to me, I just keep smiling and talking to them with a positive attitude. Eventually, they realize how easy I am to talk to and stop feeling uncomfortable. Here are a few stories from the appointment book.

꩜

Date: Monday, January 11, 2010

Time: 10:00 a.m.

Client: Celeste

Service: Color and haircut

     Celeste is always very happy when she enters the salon. Most people would call her perky. I enjoy her salon visits. She always has a great story to tell. Celeste played lead guitar for a band, and they traveled a lot. I would listen to her episodes from each performance. She was very attractive and would turn heads when she entered a room. The drummer in the band was a good friend of her husband's. She liked him a lot. This particular day, she was talking about the trip the band had just taken to another city. When they finished performing, they all went back to the drummer's room to relax. Everyone left about 1 a.m., except for Celeste. They had had a little too much to drink during the evening hours. Before they realized it, according to her story, they were in each other's arms in his hotel room. I did not have any good advice for her, except to leave her best performance on the stage. I also told her to take her husband the next time she travels with the band.

Time: 11 a.m.

Client: Bea

Service: Haircut

     Bea was a very quiet but friendly person, and we had a hard time communicating at first until she felt more comfortable with me. Bea had been married for five years but could not get pregnant for the first three years of her marriage. She loved her husband and desperately wanted to have more than one child. She told me how happy she was when she finally became pregnant with their daughter, and they were hoping for one more baby. She talked about her husband all the time. He was thoughtful and considerate, and he bought her flowers on all of their special occasions. Life was good for her.

❦

Time: 1:30

Client: Theresa

Service: Haircut

     Theresa is a loyal client. I met her about two months ago at the salon. She always has good stories to tell me about her family. These stories include going to a resort for snow skiing or to the movies.

     She never complains about all of the school activities that her children are involved in, or the guitar lessons her son takes after school. If her children called her on her cell phone, which they often did during her salon visit, she stopped everything she was involved in to answer her cell phone.

One day, Theresa came into the salon to have her hair cut and styled. Before I started her service on her hair, she showed me her watch. She was so upset because she broke it that morning, and she did not have any time to get it fixed. After we talked about how much she relies on her watch every day. She put the broken watch in her pocket and we continued to talk about her children. It was always a pleasant visit for us.

Later that same day, I started to clean my station and noticed something other than hair in the pile that I had just swept. The object I found was Theresa's watch. I picked it up and put it in my purse. I had planned to drive to her house to give it back to her later that day. I left work late and decided not to drop it off until the next day.

When I arrived home from work, my husband asked me to go to Kmart to go shopping with him. As we were shopping, I looked in my purse and noticed Theresa's broken watch in my purse. I decided to have the watch fixed for her and surprise her with it at her next appointment.

I could hardly wait for Theresa to call for her next salon appointment. Nothing makes me happier than to help a friend in need.

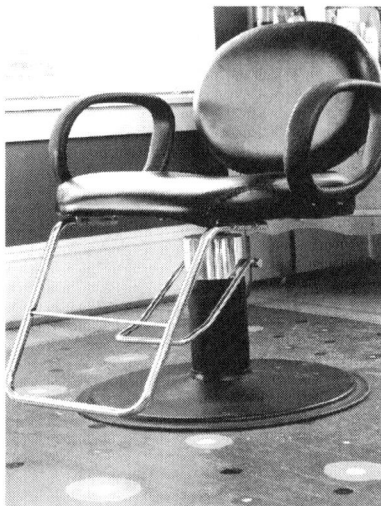

෨

Time: 2:00 p.m.

Client: Diana

Service: Color and haircut

Diana came into the salon one day with a smile on her face and a lot of energy in her spirit. We met at the health club where we both worked out. The majority of people who go to a health club on a regular basis see the same people every day. We started talking to each other and became friends.

She would talk to me about what an avid reader she had become. I heard about the many different authors who have inspired her with their writing techniques.

Diana told me that her husband was the back stage manager for a famous band. I told her I had never heard of his band; however, I was interested in stories about her husband traveling with them. She asked me if I would like to take a few of my friends to a concert to watch the band perform. After the concert we could go back stage for a meet-and-greet. The meet-and-greet sounded like a lot of fun. I was intrigued by this new experience.

I was always looking for something different to do with my friends. Diana's offer sounded like a lot of fun. I told Diana this would be a great girls' weekend retreat. My friends were happily married women and had no interest in the band members, other than earning bragging rights to say we had met members of a popular band.

♋

Date: Monday, February 22, 2010

Time: 10:00 a.m.

Client: Celeste

Service: Color and haircut

Celeste did not take the advice I had given her the last time she was at the salon. She told me she thought about me every time she looked at the drummer. It was my voice, she said, that came from the little angel on her shoulder who was telling her to stay away from him. It was hard to not be social while traveling and performing for an audience. (She could have been a great hairstylist with her social skills.)

Celeste started to talk about the drummer before she said a word about her husband. I became concerned. She acted as if she was spending more time with the band members than her family. This was unusual for her. I used to hear about the fun trips she planned to take with her husband and family. Now all I am hearing about are the fun trips with her band.

The drummer was now calling her, more than just for band practice. She would go to lunch with him at least three times a week. She admitted to enjoying the time they spent together outside of the band activities.

My advice was to find another band, or she would be sorry someday. She did not seem to care what other people thought. She did not think she was doing anything wrong. She loved her husband, but the new attention from another man was exciting for her.

I just listened and gave enough advice to make sure my client remains my client for a long time.

℧

Time: 11:00 a.m.

Client: Bea

Service: Haircut

Bea could not wait to tell me what an idiot her husband was. He would go out to the bar with his friends whenever it was convenient for him, but when she went out with her friends, he would get irate with her. She told me he would grab her by her arm and ask for every detail of her evening. She felt very threatened by his behavior. She also told me how she was afraid to come home at night after going out with her friends. She decided to just stay home and not go out with her friends anymore.

I told her that is not a good idea, he needs to let you have your own friends, and trust you when you are not with him. She started to cry and admitted to me that he would choke her and get so mad at her after she went out with her friends. She did not think it was worth ruining her marriage.

I asked her, "What marriage are you talking about? Marriages are about trust and love for each other, not one person controlling the other person." I told her she should leave the house until he treats her with the respect she deserves. If he doesn't stop now, it's only going to get worse if you have more children.

She then told me she did not want any more children because his jealous behavior started after the baby was born. She admitted to me that he would pour beer over her head as she was breast-feeding her daughter. My eyes got so big after she told me about his abusive behavior, if I had contact lenses in my eyes, they would have popped out. This type of treatment infuriates me. She is allowing this man to abuse her and her child.

You cannot make stories up like this.

Date: Tuesday, February 23, 2010

Time: 1:30 p.m.

Client: Theresa

Service: Haircut

I had been waiting for this day since Theresa's last appointment six weeks ago. I had her watch in my station with a new band on it, ready for her to wear home. I greeted her with a huge smile on my face. She looked at me as if I was going to tell her more of my great news about my life. Little did she know I was about to make her life much happier.

With my arms outstretched, hoping she would notice her watch on my wrist, I gave her a big welcoming hug. I could see a suspicious look in her eyes. She knew I was plotting something in my head. She quietly asked me what was going on before she entered the salon.

I leaned into her and said, "I have a great surprise waiting for you."

With squinting eyes, she laughed at my comment. "I know you always have some sort of surprise every time I come into see you."

I proceeded to tell her she had to figure out what the surprise was. Then she started to look around as if I was hiding a person from her. We laughed and laughed until I told her I needed to start cutting her hair, and she makes guesses about the surprise while I styled her hair.

While I was cutting her hair, I purposely waved my wrist with her watch in exaggerated gestures. She opened her mouth and put her hand over it. She proceeded to tell me that she lost a watch just like the one I had on the last time she was in the salon.

I took her watch off my wrist and handed it to her. She immediately started to cry. When I asked her why she was crying, she responded by saying that no one had ever done anything so thoughtful and nice for her.

My heart went out to her. She was married with children. She also had brothers and sisters. Why was this act of kindness so rare for her?

This small act of kindness meant a lot to Theresa. There are so many people all around us who just need a smile or a door opened for them to make them happy. It's not always the big things in life that make one person's day a little brighter, but the small simple things that you can do every day.

Time: 2:00 p.m.

Client: Diana

Service: Color and haircut

As Diana walked into the salon, she had a little sway in her walk and her face was glowing with pride. She could not wait to ask me about my girls' weekend retreat which had she set up for three of my friends and me.

"So," she asked, "how was your weekend?"

I told her it was a lot of fun. My friends and I had never met a famous band before. In fact, none of us had ever met any famous people in our lives.

I thanked her for taking care of all of the arrangements. She did an amazing job. We were booked for two nights in a local hotel, we had free buffet tickets for lunch, and she walked us right into the evening performance with front row seats to watch the band perform. After the show, Diana asked us to wear a back stage pass around our necks for security clearance to the meet-and-greet. The pass was a laminated picture of the band attached to a long thin cord with the date and location of the performance. It was a great keepsake from the occasion.

She was accustomed to making arrangements for herself and her family, so she was happy to oblige. I told her we had a blast.

Diana said, "The band members enjoyed your group of friends because you did not act like groupies. In fact, the lead singer of the band was so shocked when he sat next to you at the lounge table."

He had tried to sit next to me in Carol's chair, but I said, "Could you please find another seat? My friend was sitting there."

He looked at me and asked, "Do you know who I am?"

"Yes," I had said. I told him his name so that he'd believe me. "But you still need to find a different seat. This one's taken."

He just looked at me like he couldn't believe I was not excited that he was sitting next to me. I motioned for him to get up and sit elsewhere, so he decided to sit on my lap just to make the table laugh and it worked.

I told Diana that we sat at the table in the bar with the band members for over three hours just telling jokes and enjoying the company.

She said, "The band members are all married, and they enjoy talking to women who treat them like regular people."

"I'm sure being on the road with strangers approaching you would get old fast," I said to Diana.

"Yes it does," she replied quickly.

We continued to talk about our families, as we always did during her appointments. Diana booked her next appointment and left with a smile.

॰ঔ

Date: Monday, March 15, 2010

Time: 10:00 a.m.

Client: Celeste

Service: Color and haircut

When Celeste walks into the room, you can tell by her eyes if she has been having too much fun. Her head was tilted forward; her chin was down on her chest. Her eyes were dancing, looking up at me. I knew it was going to be an interesting day.

I asked her, "What now, my big-eyed lady?"

She laughed and told me I would not approve of her behavior. I always scolded my clients if I thought they were not being faithful to their husbands.

She told me, "Not everyone has an attentive husband like you do. You are so in love and happy with your husband that you do not even look at other men the way I do. You do not understand what I am going through."

"If you are so unhappy, then you should leave him and let him know how you feel. Do not play games behind his back," I warned her.

She did not want to hear what I had to say. She only wanted to vent to me. So I let her vent.

She said, "He is so much fun and gives me the

attention I need. I am just enjoying the day by day excitement it gives me to be with him, but I know it won't last for long."

She told me it was just too easy for them to be together because they have been friends in the band for years.

"Everyone just thinks we are practicing," she said. "If they only knew we were practicing other skills we have, they would not approve of all the time we spend together alone."

We finally started to talk about our families on a more positive stream of conversation. She left the salon with a smile on her face and she looked as if she didn't have a care in the world.

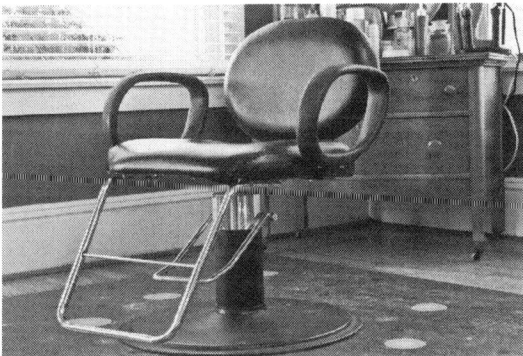

Time: 12:00 p.m.

Client: Bea

Service: Haircut

When Bea walked into the salon on this day, she was not herself. She did not make eye contact with me for a length of time. Her eyes were looking at the ground instead of looking in my eyes.

I did not continue the conversation from her last visit, even thought it was running in my head as soon as she sat down in my chair. I was thinking of what had told me because I could remember every word she had said to me. I had decided not to bring it up unless she said something first.

Bea was quiet at first, and then as she started to relax in the chair, she continued telling me her story. She asked me if I remembered her telling me how her husband had poured beer over her head while she was breast-feeding the baby. She added, "That was nothing compared to what he is doing to me now."

Bea continued to tell me how her husband had come home late from the bar and put a pillow over her face as she was sleeping. Then he would laugh as she struggled to pull it off. She could not sleep at night, in fear of what he might do to her.

If Bea tried to relax and read a book outside, her husband would walk up to the chair and flip it out from underneath her. He was becoming someone she did not know anymore. With his rude behavior, she did not want to know him. Bea knew she had to leave the man she truly loved. He was no longer the same man she had married. He thought he was so perfect for her, until the birth of their daughter. He had become very mean and unreliable.

I told her, "I have heard about husbands who change after they become a father. If men feel like you are giving the baby all of the attention they were used to getting from you, then they will resent the child. This makes the man act out in ways that he may not have prior to the baby being born."

Bea said that she tried to include her husband whenever she had the baby in her arms. She would take care of the child's needs first, and then include him in whatever she was doing afterwards. He was angry and wanted all of the attention. He wanted the attention as soon as he walked in the door from work. She was always at the door with a kiss before the baby came along, and he still expected it now.

Bea felt like she was under so much stress, trying to please her husband all the time. The baby's needs had to come first, and she felt that he needed to cope with his selfishness. Bea's husband's behavior had to change.

Bea was going to take care of her baby first. If her husband could not help her with the feedings and changing diapers, then he did not deserve to be a father. He was obviously not ready to be a parent.

Bea asked me to go to lunch with her. She offered to pay for my lunch because she was embarrassed for talking through the appointment about her horrible situation. I told her it came with the job. That was the first time I saw a smile on her face in a long time.

We went to lunch for an hour and then went our separate ways. I couldn't stop thinking about her the rest of the day. What she told me had touched me.

My husband reaped the benefits when he came home from work that evening. Listening to unhappy couples at work makes me appreciate how happy I am, realizing how lucky I was to have children who had both loving parents.

All parents should love their children, but they do not always know how to show them. I tell my family and friends that they do not love their children more than I love mine, and I do not love my children more than they love theirs. We all show affection in many different ways.

This was another day I realized not everyone is just like my family. I try to appreciate what I have, and I try not to dwell on what I don't. I pray for peace and love to all of the innocent children around the world.

෨෬

Date: Monday, April 26, 2010

Time: 10:00 a.m.

Client: Celeste

Service: Haircut

It was a gorgeous day in April. I had a gut

feeling that the clients were all going to be positive without bring drama into this sunny day.

The gorgeous part held true, but not so the day without drama. I looked at my appointment book and saw Celeste's name on my schedule. Celeste is always gorgeous but not always without drama. I never really know what she was going to talk about when she came into the salon. I always let her lead the conversation.

She told me she thought I would be happy to know she had planned on leaving the band. I was not expecting her to make this decision so soon. The last time she came into the salon, she was happy with her life, and now she was changing a very important part of it.

She finally realized what a great family she had at home. Her family needed her attention more than any of the band members needed her. She said she thought about how much time she was spending away from her family, and it wasn't what she wanted.

I asked her what the band members thought of her decision, especially the drummer. I was trying to be nosey with a little bit of class by including the other members, when I only wanted to hear the scoop on the drummer and her. She started to cry. With her whimpering voice and broken up words, she told me how difficult that decision was for her. She still had feelings for the drummer but had to let him go before those feelings ruined her family life. She continued to tell me how the drummer became almost violent towards her when she told him about her decision to leave the band. She said he grabbed her by her arm and asked her what she thought she was doing to their relationship. She had to tell him that there could no longer be a relationship between them. He then released her arm and looked at her with evil in his eyes. She said he looked like he wanted to punch something, and she was praying that it would not be her. She saw a side of him that she had never seen before. Celeste asked him to be her friend and not her lover. He told her he thought friends could become lovers but once a lover defies him, as he felt she did, he could never remain her friend. He walked out of the room and slammed the door so hard he knocked a picture off the wall.

Naturally, I consoled her and told her she was fortunate to see this evil side of him before she became too involved with him. She finally smiled and agreed with me about her decision.

I was thrilled that she had come to her senses. She made a good decision for her and her family.

※

Date: Monday, April 26, 2010

Time: 12:00 p.m.

Client: Sandy

Service: Color and haircut

My next client came into the salon with an inquisitive expression. She requested that I be her stylist. She proceeded to tell the receptionist about her friend who had had her haircut by me the previous week, and she liked her friend's results. She requested to have the same haircut as her friend.

After we discussed the haircut that Sandy requested, she started to tell me stories about her friends who would not hang out with one of her new friends because of the girl's size. She was heartbroken to watch the look on her new friend's face when other girls ignored her. She was just like the other girls inside; she just was carrying around extra weight.

Sandy was very mature for her high school age. She also did not know that she was beautiful. She had many different friends. She couldn't understand why all of them could not hang out together.

She met new friends at school and would try to include the new friend in the activities with her old friends. To her surprise, the old friends were not very cordial. They told Sandy they did not want to include her new friend because they did not think the guys would look at them if she was with them.

Sand said she told her friends that if her new friend was not invited to go out with the group, then she was not going out with them either. She went to the movies with her new friend and had a great time. The new friend was so shocked that Sandy would choose her over the other girls. She liked the new friend and did not care what her other friends thought.

Eventually Sandy was doing everything with her new friend and found herself not even including the others. The two girls were good friends for about three years until Sandy left home for college. She lost contact with the new friend until she finished college. She said she came home for a job interview and ran into her friend from high school. That was how she found out that one of the girls who would not have anything to do with the new friend years ago was now one of the girl's best friend.

Sandy said they would not have anything to do with the girl as a group, but when one of her old friends had a class with the girl, she realized how much they had in common and enjoyed many of the same movies. Her friend said she kept running into this girl at various places and they would start talking. Eventually they exchanged phone numbers and have been good friends for years now.

Sandy was so happy to hear about her new friend. She was even happier to know that the heavier girl was now accepted by her peers. The girls looked past her weight issue and saw her inner beauty.

I'm sure most of my readers have heard the phrase "nobody knows what goes on behind closed doors." When certain clients start to feel very comfortable sitting in their stylist's chair, they start to open up to them and talk about subjects they would not share with just anyone. The work done is sometimes just as much psychology as it is cosmetology. We have listened to many people with different types of personalities talk about their personal feelings. The clients vent; the stylist's console. The clients ask the stylists' opinions; the stylists oblige.

A young man came to the salon I was working in for his monthly haircut. He was always dressed like a business man and was very polite. He never talked a lot. He seemed to have a lot on his mind. On one particular visit to the salon he surprised me when he asked me if I would try to force a man to sexual harass me. I was very young at this time and just laughed at the accusation. I seriously thought he was just trying to get a reaction out of me.

He continued to tell me that I could make a lot of money if I would be willing to make this happen. Again I just laughed at his accusation because I knew I would never try to do something like that to another person. It was not appropriate.

This man never returned to the salon again. Hairstylists have many private conversations with clients on a daily basis. We need to be cautious with the conditions we are subjected to with total strangers. I realized that had I taken this conversation seriously, I could have been a victim of a crime. An innocent person could have been accused of something my client schemed. Thank God I was not a gullible person. I just said "no" and ended the conversation instantly.

Chapter **8**

Who is Worthy, Who is Not

When I became a stylist many years ago, my favorite part of the day was meeting new and interesting people. A new stylist at an established salon always waits for the walk-in clientele. This is how hairstylists build their own clientele.

This story is about a client who was very friendly, and we became friends throughout his visits. We talked about my family most of the time. He would always talk about his wife, and I would talk about my husband. I made sure I always talked about how much fun I had with my husband and children as I was cutting a male client's hair just to send the message that I was not interested in any other male relationships.

One day while I was in the backroom, I heard the front door open. I could hear a client enter the salon. Then I heard the client tell the receptionist to tell me that my secret admirer was here. I did not think anything about what he just said because I was always kidding around with my clients and assumed this person was not even aware of what he said.

I left the backroom and enter the front desk area to greet my next client. I never did tell this client that I heard him call me his secret admirer because I never really believe clients mean what they say when they are just making small talk at the receptionist desk.

We always had deep conversations about all kinds of people. We had nothing in common, and I treated this client just like I would any other client. He left the salon, and I assumed I would not see him until the next salon visit.

I cleaned my station as I always did after each client leaves my station and decided to go to lunch. When I walked to my car, my last client was standing near my car. I made small talk but continued to open the car door as to enter my car. He asked me if he could ask me a personal question that he had intended to ask me while I was styling his hair.

"What do you think about sexual threesomes?" he asked.

I stopped what I was doing and gasped for air.

"What are you talking about?" I asked, very disturbed by the question.

"Oh," he said, "don't tell me that you don't talk about threesomes with your husband. All men think about it."

"No, my husband and I have never talked about anything like that before, and I would prefer if you didn't either!" I yelled.

He tried to continue the conversation with me, but I told him I didn't have a lot of time to go out to lunch before my next client would be arriving.

He got into his car and left the parking lot. I didn't let the conversation bother me because I knew how this client liked to talk about personal situations and could get really deep into any type of subject.

I had hoped to never see this client again. I thought he would be too embarrassed to show his face in the salon again. Yet, six weeks later, he made another appointment at the salon. He did not scare me at all. I knew his wife, and he knew I could contact her at any time. During this visit he was his usual cordial self and did not ask me any inappropriate questions. We talked about my family. He always told me how he thought I was the best looking sister of the four sisters. I did not really care because I knew he was just making conversation with me. I was very relieved after he left the salon.

Weeks had gone by, and I did not see this client's name on the books. Then about eight weeks after his last visit to the salon, I received a phone call on my home phone. This was so long ago that I did not yet have a cell phone. I could not believe who was on the other end of the phone: it was one of my clients from the salon. I asked what his name was because I did not allow my clients to call me at home. When he told me who he was, I was alarmed. I asked him how he got my home phone number.

He said he saw one of my sisters at a store, and she gave it to him. He asked me if I was cutting hair in my house at all. I quickly told him that I never cut my clients' hair in my home and that he would have to make an appointment at the salon. He was very cordial, and I thought he was going to hang up the phone after I answered him.

This man continued to talk and told me he had a dream about me. I thought this was a very odd conversation between a stylist and a client, but he was a very deep person. I did not want to ask him what the dream was about, but he continued to tell me anyway. He said that he dreamed that I was cutting his hair at my house, and the more hair I cut off, the more clothes I took off.

My eyes grew wide, and my mouth opened even wider. "Well," I said, "now I know why I don't cut my clients' hair at my home."

He asked me what I thought about the dream.

"I will tell you what I think about your nasty dream. Do not bother coming into the salon for another haircut by me again." I hung the phone up on him. I was uncomfortable at home now because he had just freaked me out. I went to my sister's house until my husband came home.

As soon as my husband walked into the door, I told him what my client said to me. He was so mad about the indecent behavior that he wanted to call him and give him a piece of his mind. I calmed him down and told him I would tell my receptionist and boss not to book him for another appointment ever again. Naturally my husband told me he did not want me to go near this man ever again, and if he did approach me that I should call him right away.

Luckily for me, the receptionist told this nasty client that I would not be scheduling any haircuts with him again and he would need to go to another salon for his haircuts. He did oblige. I could not have been any happier.

There is one more little twist to this story: this man was a pastor from my church. I thought I could trust him. Just because he was a man of God did not mean he was not a human being. He did leave me alone after I ignored his calls. I have not seen or heard anything about him since that day.

People will try to enter your life, but only you can decide who is worthy and who is not.

Chapter 9

Her Pollyanna

I enjoy talking to all of my clients about their families, their jobs, and their personal feelings. The clients have to like the stylist's work in order for them to keep returning for services. When the client also likes your personality, it is an extra perk to the job. When hairstylists connect with their clients and have a bond with them, it is a great experience for both the stylist and the client.

The small talk I enjoy during a haircut service is priceless. I try to be very positive and upbeat. Most clients don't want to hear how sick you are or how miserable you feel even though they love to tell their hairstylist how sick and miserable they are. One of my most unfortunate clients was also my most memorable client.

She was a woman who had multiple sclerosis. She was a very cordial person. She started coming into the salon on her own before the multiple sclerosis took over her body. Several stylists in the salon knew her and just adored her. We slowly watched her body deteriorate. Her wonderful husband brought her into the salon to have her hair styled once a week. He never complained about the extra work she caused him. He had to bathe her and dress her daily. He even made sure that her makeup looked as if she had applied it herself. If my husband ever had to apply my make up, I'm certain that I would look more the secretary, Mimi, from *The Drew Carey Show*, than myself.

As the weeks continued to go by, she had to completely rely on others to get her through the day. She talked to me about her everyday struggles to accomplish the simple tasks in life. She slowly became weaker and weaker. I hurt my back when I tried to move her during one of her appointments; she could no longer move herself into the proper position for her shampoo. The next time, I had to ask for help to lean her head back in the shampoo bowl because I did not want to take a chance of pulling a muscle in my back again. I never let her see the strain she was causing me during her visits. It was such a pleasure to make her feel beautiful and see the joy she received from having her hair washed and styled. The visit should be all about the client and not the stylist.

Toward the end of her visits, she was not capable of even whispering her words to me. She communicated to me by nodding her head. She loved to ask me about my children when she was healthier. She would smile as I just lead her into my own personal world with my words.

She made me realize how comforting it is to hear about someone else's life when your own life is in turmoil. It was an escape for her. I could tell by the look in her eyes. She would often squeeze my hand to indicate her pleasure.

Her last nickname for me was Pollyanna. She told me I reminded her of the character Pollyanna portrayed in a book she enjoyed reading. She said Pollyanna was always happy and did nice gestures for other people, just like I did.

After we hadn't heard from her for a few weeks, I called her husband at home to find out how she was feeling. He said she did not recognize him or her own children now. With tears in my eyes, I asked him who was styling her hair for her. He said he had a nurse who visited her for hours a day, and that he was washing her hair for her. I so desperately wanted to offer my services to my friend, but I wanted to remember her as she was when I was her Pollyanna.

Chapter 10
Deal or No Deal

Hairstylists are well known to be fun and outgoing people. This trait has gotten me into a few precarious situations. One of my favorite stories involves my good friend and client, Jodie, and my youngest daughter. While Jodie was leaning back in the shampoo bowl getting her hair shampooed for her haircut, she asked me to go to a casting call to audition for the popular television game show, *Deal or No Deal*. I immediately went online to complete the requisite form in order to participate at the casting call.

The casting call was from 8:00 a.m. until 1:00 p.m. in Southfield, Michigan. My youngest daughter and I were in line by eight. We could not believe what we saw. The line was so long that we did not know if we would be able to participate in the casting call. There was an estimated one thousand people already standing in line when we arrived.

After my daughter and I stood in line for four hours, we were told that some of the people ahead of us had spent the night at the parking lot in order to be the first in line. My daughter had to go to work by 1:00, so she could not stay in line with me any longer. I was so intrigued by this casting call and really wanted to experience what it was all about. I told her to go to work and leave me there. I did not know how I was going to get home, but I was not going to go home until I had an audition.

My friend Jodie called me not more than ten minutes after my daughter left me.

"Where are you?" she asked.

"I'm about the one thousand and three hundredth person in line," I said.

Jodie walked around the circumference of the parking lot, and I jumped in the air when she would tell me which numbered light pole she was near. The people around me thought I was crazy when I just kept jumping and jumping until Jodie walked up to me, laughing hysterically.

We had so much fun looking at all of the people who dressed up for the casting call. One woman had a bald cone head on her head to imitate Howie Mandel's bald head. Many people dressed in wild colored clothes to attract the attention of the casting personnel.

We did not eat or drink anything for several hours. Finally they had a booth set up with pizza and drinks for sale. We saw people who ordered pizza from their cell phones and had it delivered through a fence.

We did not get inside the building until 5:00 p.m. Luckily, it was a gorgeous day in May. After we were inside the building, we sat in an auditorium for two more hours. The *Deal or No Deal* staff stood on a stage and gave us the instructions so we would know what to do when we walked behind the stage. Five people lined up in front of each staff member, who directed each potential contestant to talk about himself or herself for twenty seconds each. The casting directors did not want to hear how much we loved the show or Howie.

Jodie and I each had our twenty-second audition. After the other three people had their audition, the woman asked me to come back to the table. She asked me several other questions. Then she told me to walk around the corner and take a form to a man sitting at a table. We were each told to read our packet of information and go to the next audition within two days.

When I walked out of the room, the first person I saw was Jodie. She was so excited for me. We hugged each other and screamed. I do not remember Jodie driving me home because we were laughing and yelling all the way to my house.

The second audition was on a Monday at 6:00. I had to fill out several forms with many questions and information about me and my family. I was told to bring five friends and family members to a location in Southfield to audition in front of a camera. My husband had to work, so I asked my two lovely daughters, my handsome son in-law, my very cute sister, and my beautiful friend Jodie to go to the audition with me. After we waited for an hour for the second audition, we entered a room with a staff member who filmed us standing in a line just like we would stand if we were on the show. We hammed it up for the camera. The staff member constantly told us she thought we were great.

After I picked my case, the staff member stopped talking and asked my oldest daughter why she had tears in her eyes.

She said, "My mom deserves this so much."

I walked over to her and gave her a big hug.

The staff member then told us I had to pick a card from her hand. If the card said no, then I would not have a chance to appear on the show, If the card said yes, then I would have a chance to appear on the show. We all looked at each other in silence. I quickly picked a card and it said yes. The room erupted with cheers. We grabbed each other and jumped up and down.

We finally controlled our emotions and thanked the staff member for having us at the audition. As we were leaving the room my son-law asked the staff member if he could see the card in her hand which I did not chose. She would not show it to him but she smiled and winked at him. He told us later that day at our dinner celebration that the other card had yes written on it.

Sadly, the end of this story is not a call to go to California for a taping of the show. I was told that if I did not hear from the *Deal or No Deal* staff within a year, then most likely I would not make it on the show.

We were very disappointed after the year came and went, but the auditioning experience was amazing for all of us.

Chapter 11

Alone Time with the Boss

This story is a typical story that hairstylists hear from clients who own their own businesses. Sometimes it is the woman's story, and other times it is the man's story. This story is about a husband and wife who were in business together.

June and her husband owned a health club together. As husband and wife working together, they got along very well. June enjoyed working with her husband. He didn't want to hire strangers to help with the business. They tried hiring friends and family when they first started the business, but they soon found that no one works as hard as the owners do.

June did admit to getting pretty angry sometimes if her husband wouldn't take a break. He would work until the last client left. She learned to take a break when she felt like she needed one, not wait until after her husband took a break.

As the business grew, June decided to hire two assistants, one each to open and close the heath club. This gave her more flexibility since she found she was working more hours than she wanted to work. June was excited to hire more personnel to ease her workload.

June trained the new employees until she felt they were competent enough to work on their own. Now she could come and go as often as she wanted to. Life was great, and the business was doing very well.

One day when June came into the salon to have her hair cut and styled, she asked my opinion about an employee referring to herself as the girlfriend of June's husband.

"What?" I asked her. "Why would an employee have the nerve to say that to a married man?"

June said she hadn't thought anything of it at the time. She felt it was said in a fun, kidding way. The person who overheard this conversation didn't like what she heard. She told June what the employee had said because she felt it was inappropriate.

Many clients come into the salon not only for a haircut and style but for advice on their life. We are always asked what we think about a situation or what would we do if we were in the client's shoes.

I asked June to tell me the whole story.

She continued to tell me how the employees were sitting at a table with her husband getting ready to order their lunch. Her husband told them that he was told by his wife to buy their lunch on that particular day.

The new female employee looked at the waiter before she ordered, and asked him, "Isn't it nice when the wife tells her husband to buy lunch for his girlfriend?"

The waiter was as speechless as the other people at the table. June's husband, June was told to let it go right over his head.

My advice was also to let it go. If her husband did not respond, then she shouldn't either. June agreed.

I told her to make sure she keeps an eye on all of her employees. Some people will try to take her place when she is not there. They will act like they own the business and try to control situations they should not be controlling. She agreed and we quit talking about her business and just talked about our families. We enjoyed small talk for the duration of June's style appointment that day, and June left the salon in a better mood than the one she came in with.

Six weeks later, June returned for her next haircut and style. We always started our conversations with family information. We enjoyed filling each other in on our lives. Then I asked her how her health spa was doing. Her whole tone had changed in the time it took me to finish asking that short question.

She continued to tell me it was doing very well. She didn't have to go in everyday but would help her husband when he needed it. On one occasion she was working with this employee and her husband. The husband asked the two women to go to the end room and clean it for the next client. He then went to clean another room. The worker told June that she was going to help the husband, and she proceeded to follow the husband instead of going with June as she had been instructed. June said she did not really think anything of the situation because that just meant the second room would be cleaned faster with two people instead of one.

As June was working alone, one of the other employees came into the room. He asked her why she wasn't helping her husband instead of the new worker. June responded by saying she just wanted the jobs to be finished in a timely manner. She did not really care who helped her as long as the work was completed properly. June had known this worker for several years and liked his work ethic. She could tell something was bothering him. He proceeded to tell June that he and the other workers did not like how this employee was always trying to be with June's husband. He also told her he did not think that this employee was doing her job very well. According to him, this girl would be in the office or wherever June's husband would be, instead of where she needed to be to get her job done. June was shocked to hear about this kind of behavior and told the young man she appreciated his honesty and would talk to her husband about it. She told the worker to let her know any time he observed any inappropriate behavior from the girl towards her husband.

As soon as June finished her story, she asked me what I would do if I was in her shoes. I asked her if she felt uncomfortable around this person. She said she did not have a problem with her and felt comfortable around her.

We both decided June needed to just keep an eye and ear out for this worker. June told me that her husband told her everything about the workers. He even told her some of the conversations he had with this person. It was obvious to see he was very easy to talk to. All of the workers would sit in his office longer than they should. June was not threatened at all by this coworker at this time.

June returned to the salon for her six week haircut and style and was obviously annoyed at something. I asked her how she was doing that day, as I greet each client before we start his or her service.

She told me that she had been observing that female employee. She noticed how all of the other employees worked together, but this girl would only work with June's husband. Wherever he was, she would be right there, too. June was not a jealous person and trusted her husband's decisions at work. She decided to test the employee, however, by working with both of them to see how she would react.

The result? The employee treated June like a co-worker and not the owner and her employer. This girl would get things for June's husband and stand right next to him the whole day. June could not even finish asking her husband a question before the employee would answer for him. She ignored June, but she laughed and smiled with June's husband. June felt like this person was deliberately trying to exclude her. June could tell that her husband sensed her uneasy feeling because he would always come over to his wife as soon as she walked into the health spa to give her a kiss.

We decided that this worker saw how loving June and her husband were with each other, and that she must want what June had. She liked how June's husband treated his wife, and the employee wanted him to treat her with the same compassion.

I could not believe what I was hearing. I told June that I had never heard of this type of behavior from an employee when the wife is right there watching her. June was sure her husband was not even aware of this employee's intentions. He talked about the conversations the two of them had, but he never reacted to her inappropriate suggestions or comments.

June said she was just tired of all the drama. She

said her goodbyes and would keep me informed at her next visit in six weeks.

June always kept her word, and six weeks later, she returned for her haircut with another story about her annoying employee. She didn't even explain to me what we were going to do to her hair before she started talking angrily.

One day, June walked into the office, and her husband asked her to look at the e-mail he just received from one of the employees. June read the e-mail and noticed it was about more than work. The author of the email message complimented June's husband about how he looked that day in his blue shirt. The message went on to ask if he was relaxing at home and having a martini yet.

There were several other e-mails from this same person. June only read the one e-mail her husband asked her to read. She told me she decided later that day to read all the e-mails from this person and wonder why she never mention June's name when she really should have included her in the conversation.

The only advice I could give June was to tell her husband that she didn't like what she was reading in the e-mails that he was getting from one of his employees. He needed to talk to the employee. This person sounded very lonely and obviously enjoyed June's husband's company and attention.

June said her husband receives e-mail from several females. "I never feel like I need to read all of them," she explained. In fact, her husband is always asking her to read the important messages. She asked her husband if he thought any of the workers were e-mailing him about anything more than they needed to. Of course he didn't see anything wrong with employees sending him messages every day. June could not understand why they needed to e-mail when they see him at work and could ask him the same questions while they were there.

My advice to June was to tell her husband that she was going to start reading all of the e-mail to better her knowledge of the way the heath club was operating. She agreed with me, and then we changed the subject to talk about our families. June left the salon in a much better mood than one she came in with.

I enjoy the feeling I get when a client leaves the salon looking good on the outside and feeling even better on the inside.

June was the last client on my schedule that day, so I started to clean my station area before leaving for the day. I heard the salon door open and saw June returning. I asked her if she left something at my station.

"No," she replied. "I did not leave anything at your station. I just wanted to ask you about a situation I had at work."

I put my broom down and asked her to sit next to me and tell me what was on her mind.

She was concerned about two employees at work who pulled her into the office because they did not like the behavior of another co-worker. June could not believe that this was the same woman that she had just vented to me about.

The employees were all in the lunch room at work eating lunch with June's husband. They continued to tell her about her husband leaving the room to answer a phone call. He just left the room and the new employee started to wrap June's husband's sandwich with foil. Then she put all of his lunch back into the refrigerator. The other employees could not believe their eyes. They asked her why she was touching her boss's food. They told her he obviously was not finished eating his lunch. She was not eating her lunch at the time and told them he could finish eating with her after he answered his phone call. They all looked at each other. One of the employees asked her why she was always sucking up to the boss. They did not expect the answer they received. She told them she liked eating lunch with him because he treated her nicer than her own husband did. At the same time two of the employees told her he was happily married and did not need or want a girlfriend at work. She chuckled at the response and said she did not like his wife and did not care what his wife thought about her.

I was so shocked by this whole conversation that I could not say a word. I just let June vent as all good hairstylists should do.

The new employee told the co-workers that June's husband was clueless about the girl's intentions. When they were eating lunch together the other day, she asked him what he thought about affairs, because she knew a friend who was thinking about having one. He did not answer the question as if he wasn't really listening to what she had to say.

The other employees told her that the boss is always nice to all of his employees. They continued to tell her that she was getting the wrong impression from him if she thought he was personally interested in her.

"June," I raised my voice at her because I thought she was starting to let this women get to her. "I have heard a lot of stories just like this one. This woman is a lonely person who isn't use to getting male attention. You know your husband is clueless to her intentions. If your husband was interested in having an affair with this woman, he would not tell you what she talks about. You would be the last person he would confide in. He is not interested in her."

June said that she was not worried about her husband at all. She just needed to vent to me about this employee's behavior because the other workers were always telling her that this person was not doing her job as well as she should because she was spending too much time talking to June's husband.

As June talked through the situation, she decided to talk to the employee about what she was doing wrong. This would be the best way to handle the situation. After she confronted the employee, June said she didn't have any problems with the girl again. She did her job and kept to herself. The health spa was once again a pleasant place to work.

I like to give my clients positive encouragement to solve the problems they share with me. She said she liked my honest decision and never would have thought about an employee trying to ignore her in order to get closer to her husband.

The moral of this story is to keep your friends close, but keep your employees even closer.

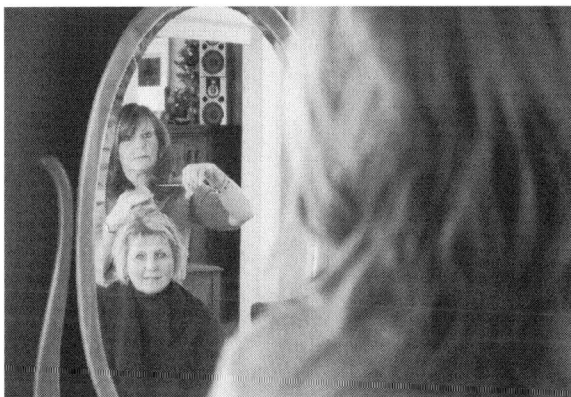

About the Author

I have been a hairstylist for over thirty years. I am married to a wonderful man. I am sure all of the authors talk about their spouses as if they are the best spouse in the world. We have to say that because our spouses are also our proofreaders. After thirty-two years of marriage, my husband still wants a kiss in the morning before I leave for work and another kiss before I say good night. We have mutual respect for each other. We call each other throughout the day to keep in touch. This is how I make sure I am always on his mind, not to mention on his cell phone. Just like my profession, my personal life revolves around communication.

We have two beautiful daughters. We are very proud of them. They have made our marriage a solid and very happy one. Our family is everything to us. We also have a son-in-law who we adore. Our daughter and son-in law blessed us with a granddaughter on July 29, 2010. They named her Brooklyn Emma. She is our world.

People have asked me what inspired me to write a book. The answer is Oprah. I watch Oprah all the time. I enjoy the stories her guests tell the world. Her show is very informative about the lives of real people. The famous entertainers on her show seem just like normal people when she talks to them. Oprah relates to every guest as if that person is her good friend.

I believe she makes people feel comfortable around her. She does not care if they are famous or an average Joe from Idaho; they are welcomed with warmth and respect on her show. Her audience has a chance to hear about famous people and their normality in their individual lives. Many shows are entertaining and educational at the same time.

My sister, Jackie Horton, has watched every show since the beginning of Oprah's career on television. I used to tell her that she had an Oprah education because she started her sentences with "Oprah said…" whenever we would talk to each other.

Penelope Cruz was a guest on Oprah's show in December 2009. Oprah asked Penelope what inspired her to become an actor. Penelope told her that her mother was a hairstylist who owned a salon when she was a little girl. Penelope would go to the salon after school and listen to all the stories the clients would talk about. Penelope also talked about how she would pretend to be doing her homework, but she was actually listening to the clients talking about their lives.

We live in Michigan. I have lived in Michigan all of my life. My new passion in life is to become a successful writer. Look for my next book about different hairstylists from Michigan.

Acknowledgments

Roxanne Gill
Stephanie Gagleard, photographer
Nicole Rodgers, illustrator

Laura
you are my
first book sale.
Thank you for all
the great conversations
everyday! Judy

Made in the USA
Charleston, SC
18 January 2011